VIAGRA

The complete guide on how to use Viagra medication to get and keep an erection to make you last longer in bed if you're finding it difficult to stay erect during sex

Dr. Lewis Jack

Table of Contents

CHAPTER 1

INTRODUCTION: UNLOCKING THE SECRETS OF VIAGRA

In the realm of medical breakthroughs, few innovations have had as profound an impact on the lives of individuals as Viagra. This small blue pill, initially designed to address the challenges of erectile dysfunction, has become a symbol of hope, transformation, and a renewed sense of intimacy for countless men around the world.

As we embark on this journey into the world of Viagra, it is essential to recognize the historical context that led to the development of this groundbreaking medication. Erectile dysfunction, a condition that has affected men throughout history, was often shrouded in silence and stigma. The quest for a solution to this deeply personal issue prompted researchers and scientists to explore new avenues of medical science, ultimately culminating in the discovery of sildenafil citrate, the active ingredient in Viagra.

This book seeks to unravel the mysteries surrounding Viagra, providing a comprehensive guide that goes beyond the surface-level understanding. We delve into the science behind this medication, exploring how it works on a physiological level and its impact on various aspects of men's health.

However, our exploration extends beyond the pharmacological aspects. We will also address the broader implications of Viagra on relationships, self-esteem, and quality of life. As we navigate the chapters ahead, we will encounter the benefits and potential risks associated with Viagra, exploring its applications beyond erectile dysfunction, and considering the lifestyle and psychological factors that play a crucial role in men's sexual health.

This book is not just a scientific exploration; it is a holistic guide intended to empower individuals with knowledge. We will debunk myths, challenge misconceptions, and provide insights into the future of erectile dysfunction treatments. Moreover, we aim to foster open conversations about men's health, encouraging a proactive and informed approach to well-being.

Whether you are someone directly impacted by erectile dysfunction, a healthcare professional seeking a deeper understanding of treatment options, or simply a curious reader interested in the intersection of science and human experience, "Viagra Unveiled" invites you to embark on a journey of discovery and enlightenment. Together, let us unravel the layers of knowledge surrounding Viagra and, in doing so, contribute to a more informed, compassionate, and empowered approach to men's health.

CHAPTER 2

THE SCIENCE BEHIND VIAGRA

Understanding the inner workings of Viagra requires a journey into the intricate landscape of human physiology and the fascinating interplay of biochemical processes. This chapter aims to demystify the science behind Viagra, shedding light on how this pharmaceutical marvel achieves its remarkable effects.

2.1 How Viagra Works

At the heart of Viagra's efficacy lies its ability to address the root cause of erectile dysfunction. This section delves into the mechanism of action, revealing the orchestrated dance of molecules within the body.

2.1.1 Mechanism of Action:

Unraveling the Role of Nitric Oxide: Explore the pivotal role of nitric oxide in the vascular system and how Viagra amplifies its effects.

Relaxation of Smooth Muscle: Understand how Viagra facilitates the relaxation of penile smooth muscle, a crucial step in achieving and maintaining an erection.

2.1.2 Nitric Oxide and its Role:

Nitric Oxide as a Vasodilator: Examine the vasodilatory properties of nitric oxide and its impact on blood flow.

Endothelial Function: Explore the intricate relationship between nitric oxide, endothelial function, and the regulation of vascular tone.

2.2 Development and Discovery

The journey to the creation of Viagra was marked by scientific curiosity, serendipity, and rigorous research. This section provides a historical overview of the milestones that led to the development of this groundbreaking medication.

2.2.1 Historical Milestones:

Early Explorations: Trace the initial investigations into vasodilators and their potential applications in treating cardiovascular conditions.

Sildenafil Citrate Discovery: Uncover the serendipitous discovery of sildenafil citrate's potential role in treating erectile dysfunction.

2.2.2 Clinical Trials and Regulatory Approval:

Rigorous Testing: Explore the pivotal clinical trials that assessed the safety and efficacy of Viagra.

Regulatory Hurdles: Navigate the regulatory landscape that Viagra traversed on its path to becoming a globally recognized treatment.

By the end of this chapter, readers will have gained a deeper appreciation for the intricate science that underpins Viagra's ability to restore not just physical function but also a sense of normalcy and confidence in the lives of those grappling with erectile dysfunction.

CHAPTER 3

UNDERSTANDING ERECTILE DYSFUNCTION

Erectile dysfunction (ED) is a complex and often misunderstood condition that transcends the physical aspects of sexual health, reaching into the emotional and psychological realms. This chapter serves as a foundational exploration, dissecting the various facets of erectile dysfunction to provide a comprehensive understanding.

Defining Erectile Dysfunction

The Anatomy of Erection:

Delve into the physiological processes that contribute to a normal erection, exploring the role of blood flow, nerve signals, and the intricate coordination of vascular and neural systems.

Understand the distinction between occasional difficulties and persistent challenges, establishing the criteria for diagnosing erectile dysfunction.

The Psychological Impact:

Examine the emotional toll of erectile dysfunction, shedding light on the potential impact on self-esteem, relationships, and overall well-being.

Addressing Stigma: Explore societal perceptions and misconceptions surrounding ED, aiming to dismantle stigma and foster open conversations.

Causes and Risk Factors

Understanding the root causes of erectile dysfunction is pivotal in tailoring effective treatments. This section delves into the multifaceted factors contributing to ED.

Physical Factors:

Vascular Health: Investigate the role of cardiovascular conditions, atherosclerosis, and hypertension in compromising blood flow to the penis.

Neurological Influences: Explore how conditions affecting the nervous system, such as diabetes and multiple sclerosis, can contribute to ED.

Psychological Factors:

Stress and Anxiety: Analyze the impact of psychological stressors on sexual performance and the development of ED.

Depression and Mental Health: Uncover the intricate connection between mental health disorders and erectile dysfunction.

Lifestyle Factors:

Smoking and Substance Abuse: Examine the effects of tobacco, alcohol, and illicit substances on sexual function.

Sedentary Lifestyle and Obesity: Investigate the correlation between physical inactivity, obesity, and the risk of developing ED.

By the conclusion of this chapter, readers will have a nuanced understanding of the physiological and psychological intricacies of erectile dysfunction, paving the way for an informed exploration of treatments and interventions in subsequent sections of the book.

CHAPTER 4

THE BENEFITS AND RISKS OF VIAGRA

Viagra, hailed as a revolutionary solution for erectile dysfunction, offers a ray of hope for individuals seeking to reclaim their intimate lives. However, like any medical intervention, it comes with a spectrum of benefits and risks. This chapter meticulously examines the positive outcomes and potential drawbacks associated with the use of Viagra.

Rapid Onset of Action:

Explore the quick onset of Viagra's effects, providing a timeline for when individuals can expect improvements in erectile function.

Understand the factors that may influence the speed at which Viagra takes effect.

Increased Confidence and Sexual Satisfaction:

Examine the psychological impact of Viagra on individuals, including enhanced confidence, reduced anxiety, and an overall improvement in sexual satisfaction.

Real-life Testimonials: Share experiences and anecdotes from individuals who have benefited from Viagra to illustrate its positive impact.

Common Side Effects:

Detail common and typically mild side effects such as headaches, facial flushing, and indigestion.

Strategies for Minimizing Discomfort: Offer practical tips for managing and mitigating common side effects.

Rare but Serious Side Effects:

Discuss infrequent but potentially severe side effects, including vision changes and priapism.

Emphasize the importance of seeking prompt medical attention in the event of serious side effects.

Viagra and Cardiovascular Health

Considerations for Individuals with Cardiovascular Conditions:

Explore the interplay between Viagra and cardiovascular health, addressing concerns and precautions for individuals with pre-existing heart conditions.

Collaboration with Healthcare Providers: Emphasize the necessity of open communication between patients and healthcare professionals to ensure safe use.

Interactions with Other Medications

Provide a comprehensive overview of medications that may interact with Viagra, potentially leading to adverse effects.

Guidance on Medication Management: Offer insights into how individuals can navigate medication interactions under the supervision of healthcare providers.

By the end of this chapter, readers will have a nuanced understanding of both the positive and potential adverse effects of Viagra, empowering them to make informed decisions about its use in consultation with healthcare professionals.

CHAPTER 5

VIAGRA DOSAGE AND ADMINISTRATION

The effectiveness of Viagra lies not just in its formulation but also in the precise dosage and administration. This chapter navigates the nuances of finding the right dosage, understanding the principles behind its administration, and ensuring optimal outcomes for individuals seeking relief from erectile dysfunction.

Initial Dosage Recommendations:

Detail the standard starting dosage for Viagra and the considerations that may influence a healthcare provider's decision.

Individualized Approaches: Discuss the importance of personalized dosage adjustments based on factors such as age, overall health, and the severity of erectile dysfunction.

Adjusting Dosage for Optimal Results:

Explore the potential need for dosage adjustments over time, considering changes in health status or treatment response.

Monitoring Side Effects: Provide guidance on how healthcare providers and individuals can collaboratively assess the need for dosage modifications based on observed side effects.

Timing of Administration:

Discuss the optimal timing of Viagra intake in relation to anticipated sexual activity.

Food Interactions: Address the influence of meals on the absorption and effectiveness of Viagra.

Lifestyle Considerations:

Explore how lifestyle factors, such as alcohol consumption and tobacco use, can impact the efficacy of Viagra.

The Role of Stress: Discuss the potential influence of stress and anxiety on the response to Viagra and strategies for mitigating these factors.

Potential Interactions with Other Substances:

Provide a comprehensive overview of substances, including certain medications, that may interact with Viagra and impact its effectiveness.

Cautionary Measures: Emphasize the importance of communicating all current medications and substances to healthcare providers to ensure safe administration.

By the conclusion of this chapter, readers will have a thorough understanding of the dosage considerations and best practices for administering Viagra. This knowledge serves as a critical foundation for individuals and healthcare providers alike, ensuring that the benefits of Viagra are maximized while minimizing potential risks and complications.

CONCLUSION: NAVIGATING THE PATH TO INTIMATE WELLNESS

As we bring our exploration of Viagra to a close, it becomes evident that this small blue pill transcends its pharmaceutical nature. It symbolizes not only a breakthrough in the treatment of erectile dysfunction but also a gateway to renewed confidence, connection, and understanding within the realm of intimate wellness.

Recap of Key Takeaways

Holistic Approach to Men's Health:

Reflect on the importance of viewing erectile dysfunction within the broader context of men's health, emphasizing the interconnectedness of physical, psychological, and emotional well-being.

Advocate for holistic approaches that consider lifestyle modifications, communication strategies, and the integration of medical interventions.

Viagra's Impact on Relationships:

Highlight the positive impact of Viagra on relationships, emphasizing the potential for improved communication, intimacy, and overall relationship satisfaction.

Acknowledge the importance of open dialogue between partners, fostering an environment of understanding and support.

10.2 Encouraging a Holistic Approach to Men's Health

Dismantling Stigma:

Revisit the societal stigmas surrounding erectile dysfunction and reiterate the importance of dispelling myths and misconceptions.

Advocate for open conversations that reduce shame and encourage individuals to seek help without hesitation.

Empowering Informed Decision-Making:

Stress the significance of informed decision-making in collaboration with healthcare professionals when considering Viagra or alternative treatments.

Encourage ongoing communication between individuals and healthcare providers to optimize treatment plans.

In concluding our journey through the intricate landscape of Viagra, we recognize that the quest for intimate wellness is multifaceted. It involves not just the pharmacological aspects of a medication but a comprehensive understanding of the individual, their relationships, and the factors influencing their overall well-being.

This book seeks to empower readers with knowledge, fostering a proactive and informed approach to men's health. Whether you are an individual navigating the complexities of erectile dysfunction, a partner seeking to understand and support, or a healthcare professional guiding patients through treatment options, may this exploration serve as a beacon of enlightenment on the path to intimate wellness.

As we step away from these pages, may the insights gained pave the way for empowered choices, fulfilling relationships, and a broader conversation that destigmatizes and embraces the diverse aspects of men's health.

THE END

Printed in Great Britain
by Amazon

37725969R00020